My life with stoma

My new life begins

Edition 3. Part 1/August 2019

J.R Lucas Wolf

Content

Table of Contents...2

Foreword..4

Introduction..9

Chapter 1. Operation...14

Chapter 2. The time after the hospital

stay...25

Chapter 3. What's a stoma?.......................................37

Chapter 4. The stoma care and the

Ileostoma..44

Chapter 5. Partnership, Family and

Friends..51

Bottom Line..62

Acknowledgements.......................................64

Bibliography...67

Imprint..69

3

Foreword

"Why am I writing this book?"
Well I think I have the right and the duty to write this book. Finally, my own person was diagnosed with Crohn's disease exactly 17 years ago. With my book I want to help other people and show them what I had to suffer from Crohn's disease. With this book I can help you to cope better with this disease.

The diagnosis was and still is terrible for me, but I have learned to live with my disease. A disease that cannot be cured today, but where the symptoms can be alleviated. After such a diagnosis one is first shocked and after a time of reflection, dejected. An enormous amount of time passes until our brain understands what is actually happening to us. Fear, anger and depression alternate.

It should also be mentioned that I was caught at a time when I was simply not expecting it in this way. It also hit me particularly hard, with Crohn's disease being classified in three categories. To my regret, the highest level was three.

For people who end up in level one, for example, the disease is a bit more harmless. With me, but the disease struck mercilessly and I almost died of it. It also hit me completely unprepared. In addition, I had never heard anything about Crohn's disease before in my life

or had read. Also I did not have any previous knowledge or experience how one behaved with this illness. That is also one of the reasons why it could hit me so hard. Mine Person made a lot of mistakes while this disease only forgives a few mistakes.

One more reason for me to write this book later. The book is structured like an encyclopedia or a Bible, where you simply look up everything you urgently need. In my book there is a lot in it that you will need every day. Everything that was not accessible to my own person, but he still needed.The book would open my eyes and I would not make one or the other big mistake anymore.Another big advantage for you as a future patient will be to be familiar with the possible forms of therapy and medication. No matter which stage of the disease you end up with, you can and will cope with Crohn's disease.

At this point we would like to say that you should take every help that is offered to you. Deal with the disease openly from the very beginning, you'll see that makes things a lot easier. Hiding won't help, but dealing with the disease will. Try to listen to your body more often.

The many signals the body sends you afterwards also to interpret correctly.

Also, pain always has a cause, ignoring it in this case only brings longer to expose the pain. Pain killers can only alleviate the pain, but not permanently fight it, or even eliminate it. The less painkillers or medications you need, the more you become less dependent on it, too. In addition, medications can be taken after a longer intake, deny the desired effect. Furthermore, there is a risk of becoming dependent on the medication if it is taken for a longer period of time.

Therefore, you should only take the medication when you really need it, and beyond that, they should also help.

Introduction

Hello, my name is J.R. Lucas Wolf and I have Crohn's disease. I had my first contact with a stoma, also called anus praeta, in December 2003.

My person was diagnosed after severe pain in the anal area, bloody diarrhea, high inflammatory values, and an unwanted anus in the abdomen. I was admitted to a nearby hospital (Bad Waldsee). Also nobody really knew what was going on with me.

My humble self had been in a rehabilitation clinic for 10 days and was now driven to the hospital with severe pain. In order to be brought afterwards to a surgeon to will be. It was immediately clear that my person had to go to a special clinic for Crohn's disease patients.

So back in the ambulance again, and quickly to the special clinic for Crohn's disease patients.

Arrived there in the special clinic, the search began. Searching for the cause of this severe pain.

I presented my findings to the doctor on duty. These findings were inadequate and outdated, so I was told that I would do all the examinations again. But first the most important of all examinations was ordered for me.

The colonoscopy also called. This colonoscopy should be carried out in the following days. First, however, a sonography (ultrasound examination) was performed, by the to the doctor on duty. Immediately after the sonography, I was admitted to the normal ward.

The first night was very restless and the next day we were woken up very early, around 7.00 o'clock. Several smaller examinations were scheduled. However, the first day was still relatively quiet.

What changed two days later was the colonoscopy. It was already my third and I had not exactly good experiences with it, in the recent past made. Accordingly my worries and excitement were big.

Immediately in the morning, after a short preparation, I was brought to the colonoscopy. Also the anesthesia should be done very quickly on my person, so that he got a film break and woke up 90 minutes later. My first question to the nurse was:

"What happened?", "And where am I?"

The nurse answered: "You're in the recovery room and you'll be taken right back to normal ward."

After my person was back in normal ward, thequestions started again. My humble self absolutely wanted to know if and when he was allowed to eat something again. Of course also how the colonoscopy had gone.

We only learned what was wrong with him in the afternoon, when he was taken to the chief physician. That one absolutely wanted to examine unserins. During the examination between the chief physician

and me, to a very serious conversation. The chief physician examined me and then discussed the next steps with me.

The doctor was also very kind to me and also tried to teach him gently.

As far as I was concerned, I was to be operated in the next few days. The pain that my own person felt caused two fistulas. In addition the intestine was very inflamed and one wanted to spare this inflamed intestine.

Chapter 1.

The chief physician wanted to remove the unwanted anus and at the same time close the fistulas in the abdomen and anal area in an operation planned especially for me. Afterwards a small intestinal outlet (Ilestoma) should be put to me.

They weren't such good news and I filled up accordingly. The chief physician tried to calm me down a bit and told me that one could also get very old with a small intestine exit.

After this conversation I was first brought back to my room.

My person should be able to cope with the operationand in the next few hours, give our written consent. What a big shock for me, that was really strong tobacco.

"How does one feel after such negative news? and after such perspectives?

Now for me, the world as he knew it came to an end. And he only wanted his peace. My ego played many scenarios through which spoke for and against an operation.

But the worst part was that nobody could really help me with my decision. My ego was now in demand and had to make the difficult decision alone.

After a very restless and almost sleepless night I woke up the following morning. It was the day of the decision for me. The decision was in and of itself, already fallen.

My ego secretly knew that too. My ego did not want a life with two fistulas and an unwanted anus!

In the course of the day, however, I signed the documents for the operations.

In the following days my own person had to undergo several preliminary examinations. In the end, the day arrived that everything should change.

Ours was brought to the operating theatre early in the morning. The chief physician himself was to perform this operation. Also this time the anaesthesia went relatively fast. My humble self was once again torn apart and woke up later in the intensive care unit. I immediately asked the first nurse I saw:

"How did my surgery go?", "and now do I have an anus?"

She answered:

"Your surgery went well and yes, you now have an anus on the right side (ileostoma)."
Thank you", I said to her.

All right, I thought to myself, at least you survived that until here! My guy was in pain and also felt the bag from the anus, on his skin. Immediately my humble self asked the nurse for some stronger painkillers. She then increased the dose.

After less than a quarter of an hour I noticed that the pain was subsiding again. My ego absolutely wanted to know what the stomach looked like, so he put the blanket aside a little gently. Oh, that really didn't look great, and all you could see everywhere were clamps and scars. What a shock me! I was just 38 years old and had a bag on my stomach for an indefinite period of time. Life as my own person knew it was over for now.

"Who would like to have someone with a bag to a friend or as a man?"

"Can you live normally with a bag," I asked myself.

"What can you do with it at all?"

It is hard to imagine what kind of impossible and negative thoughts my person had. In addition, my own person was very weak, and was also powerfully under the influence of medication. And yet she (her own person) only wanted to cry.

I just kept asking myself:

"Why only me?", "and why right now?"

But in the end it occurred to me again, I have a family and I'm loved too. My life companion (K), my brothers and sisters (A, R, G, S), and my parents, made themselves surely mightily worried about me.

After a telephone call with my partner(K), this should change a little. My person was finally happy to hear a familiar voice and, moreover, happy to hear some encouraging words. The phone call calmed me down a little, but now I was in more pain again.

So my humble self demanded another higher dose of painkillers. After taking the painkillers, Ourselves fell asleep, immediately peacefully.

Thanks to the painkillers received, my person spent a very quiet night.

In the following days I got a stomatotherapist, because I had to deal with I was supposed to learn from a stoma.

That refused my Ego but categorical. He was still not ready to deal with this topic.

A few weeks passed until my own person could slowly become friends with the thoughts, later with an anus, to be able to lead a completely "normal" life.

My humble self had gained some weight and the circulation was more stable again.

Since suddenly the next bad news camethrough the door. One of the nurses walked into the room and said to me: "Unfortunately, we have to quarantine you, you have staph."

"What are staphylococci again", I asked myself!

Now in the present my person would explain it that way: As staphylococci a spherical bacterium. These bacteria live on the skin and mucous membranes and are often harmless. However, they can also cause infections in soft tissues and internal organs, and then become life-threatening.

I did not have this information at that time. My humble self only learned that he had to lie alone in his room for a limited period of time and was not allowed to receive any visitors. Such a message would throw almost everyone off track, and with me it was no different.

But a few days later I should receive a big

surprise. My mother, my brother and my partner would visit me.

When they finally came through the door days later, I wondered what they were wearing! They were all covered in a blue coat, were wearing in addition gloves and the prescribed mouthguard. Of course it didn't look very nice, but it was very effective. Due to my weak immune system, any further infection had to be avoided. There was still a acute risk of infection, and my family also wanted not to infect me. It should also be mentioned that we had a good time anyway. In addition it became still another very beautiful day, despite this small "mask" campaign.

But when the family returned home the next day, my ego had at least filled a little hope.

You can anticipate it at this point, thestaphylococci have got rid of Us again. Physical weakness and pain partly also.

At the end, after about three months in hospital, I was released from the hospital one day.

I was put into a patient transporter and then driven home (NRW). Also it is hard to believe how long, three months can occur. In addition, my ego often thought that he would not make it anymore.

My person was emaciated to less than 50 kilograms, and that at 1.80m height. Finally, after more than three months at home again. But my person was a nursing case and therefore also in need of care.

Believe it or not, my partner(K) was really looking forward to me. Since we are both very close to the water, we first let one or two tears run together. Thereby we talked for a long time. In addition, we approved ourselves, the one or other endorphins. These are created, for example, when you snog or cuddle for a long time.

In the following days we both had a lot to discuss. In addition, a nursing service should (had to) be ordered, and a lot of other things should be done or procured.

Things like: The health insurance company, the medical supply store, the bank, etc. In addition there was a lot of paperwork to be done.

Chapter 2.

The time after the hospital stay, and here especially the first days of the change, were very difficult. Such an anus exit is not always tight, and a nursing service needs some time until it is on site.

At my little, on one or the other day, the nerves were sparkling clean. My ego still didn't want to deal with the subject of stoma.

In addition if the stoma was once leaky, I stuck inevitably simply a compress on it. My own person was bedridden and could only move with the help of a rollator.

Ours got help washing, take a shower and get dressed. I could eat alone, but I couldn't cook yet. I didn't have to stick to a special diet, butmy diet was a bit limited. Foods that caused flatulence, diarrhoea, and therefore some pain, were immediately banned from my diet.

My humble self also had a lactose-free and low-fibre diet. In addition my inflammation values were still high and so I had to omit one or the other food from my diet.

My own person had a long list of medications which had to be shortened.

But first I had to visit my gastroenterologist. But he should be delayed by a few weeks. At least until the day I regained full transportability.

Also the first visit to my gastroenterologist, as very difficult to describe, related to my stoma. The system that my person had was suboptimal and leaking more often than allowed.

On this day the acid under my skin burned. The doctor examined me and took a closer look at my stoma. On the same day my doctor gave me lots of tips and advice. Of course, regarding the handling of a stoma and the new medications she kindly prescribed for me.

My person received cortisone therapy and an antibiotic for a few weeks.

I also talked about a possible therapy with Humira, that was the name of the drug. It is a so-called immunosuppressant. This medicine is simply added to suppress the immune system. Because my own person was diagnosed with Crohn's disease and the immune system had to be suppressed. That was the only real drug for it.

But since my stoma was already pinching and I already saw the problems coming towards me, I decided to end my visit to my doctor immediately. Also on that day my person received a lot of new information and was a bit annoyed. Certainly because of the stoma that was now leaking. The whole thing was tiring and irritated my own person even more. So we drove home to order the nursing service afterwards. Our person still couldn't look at the intestine, and he couldn't change the plate, not even yet.

The bag was supposed to be delivered quite late that day.

The nursing service had taken a little more time. The nursing service responsible for me was otherwise quite fast. Also the women of the nursing service were always very nice to me, and in addition still very diligently.

I didn't get along well with my ostomy system, a visit to the medical supply store was supposed to change that.

Unserins had a good stomatotherapist in a medical supply store who helped you very well with the stoma. After we were given a different system, with a slightly larger bag and the corresponding abdominal belt, the situation changed. The new system was good to use and it didn't leak so often anymore. Another advantage was the large capacity of the new bag, which allowed me to sleep better at night. Also, the bag didn't fill so quickly anymore, and so I got to sleep at night.

A bag of overcrowded food.
Eventually, after many months in the country, Ourselves started to change the base plate and the bag.

One day the bag was leaking again and it had to be handled quickly. Ourins had a few appointments with the doctors that day and was determined to keep them. So he decided in case of an accident (Malör) to change the base plate and the bag himself.

It is difficult to overcome oneself and it requires a lot of courage, even a little overcoming. But on that day I managed all this myself and I managed it. It cost me a great deal of effort, but I was able to keep all my appointments. My ego now celebrated what is called an experience of success and that he needed it in that situation, too.

My humble self was not trained to cut and glue base plates, but he had copied it from the nursing staff. Also the base plate was not perfect and did not hold it as long as the memories last.

Normally a base plate lasted two days. It depended on how long you sat, ran, ran, showered, ate, drank and how much you sweated. Strictly speaking, such a change of base plates is not predictable or even calculable. If Unsereins tells you, for example, that the base plate always broke when you

needed it the least. You won't lose that or even believe it. But it actually always happened the same way.

It's in the nature of things, you just don't look at the base plate every five minutes, or bags. Afterwards you leave the house once and then notice that an accident (Malör) happens.

At this moment, however, it is usually already too late. Therefore I got myself a small backpack and equipped it with everything I needed to change the stoma system.

The other problem was soon to find a suitable

place (toilet) to "repair" the stoma system

My own person, as a precaution, has arranged some toilet places in the course of the time, where he could repair the bag or the base plate afterwards in peace. It should be mentioned at this point that my humble self always got a small crisis if these toilets were either occupied, defective, or there was no toilet paper left.

Strictly speaking, it really got on my nerves and today there is still something like a cleaning stick in my person.

The reason for this is that you have a weak immune system yourself, which means that an infection can quickly develop.

As a small precaution, Unserins always carried cleaning cloths with him to clean contaminated surfaces if necessary. The worst thing about my story was that the stoma seemed invisible to everyone, but the physical weakness was visible to everyone.

My own person cannot tell how many people (people) felt sorry for him, but there must have been some.

The physical weakness and the high dose of medication made us lack concentration and strength. But very few will be able to imagine what we were doing in these difficult times, I've really been through. A body that changed completely, had no more power to do so, and also the resulting not acceptance of others.

It took a few months to really cope with this new situation. Also to trust his body halfway again. Soon after that he had to slowly fight his way up from the bottom and with all the resistance not to give up frivolously. These I give simply times on thoughts, came always only then, if nothing at all more went. A strong mind cannot become happy in a weak body in the long run. Since mind and body normally form a unity, one is completely lost when one of them can no longer function or functions properly. To always be dependent on others and not be able to do anything yourself, is a total blow to one's head. This helplessness and the dependence connected with it is unbearable for my ego. We've arranged to have the stoma for a period of nine years.

Much later with his gastroenterologist after 9 years of suffering, with a stoma, decided to make an attempt. At this point it is explained that there was no other way. My person now had four fistulas around the stoma, which were also very painful and extremely dangerous.
Therefore our fistulas should be operated and at the same time the anus should be moved back.

The decision to do so was not easy. My own person, cannot say exactly how many conversations with physicians were led, until finally my person, for the I decided to do thesurgery. Just the thought of not having any more pain or stoma led to this positive

decision. The time with stoma and fistulas was almost unbearable. Without these damned (evil) fistulas it might have been bearable.

The problem with myself was that we couldn't see a hospital anymore.In addition, there was a certain amount of fear of the upcoming operation. It was just another "attempt" to change my life. It can be anticipated at this point, Ourselves underwent this operation and everything went well. The fistulas and the anus are now gone and belong to the past. The most important thing at the end: 17 years later and I have no intestinal outlet (Ileostoma) any more, and weigh again whole 76,50kg.

Here at this point ends my own story for today, but then follow many tips and some explanations, around the big topics stoma and nutrition.

Chapter 3.

I'm sure you're wondering now:

"What is a stoma or (Ileostoma)?"

Well, that's not that easy to explain. I'll try it this way:

The term "stoma" comes from Greek and means "mouth" or "opening.

A stoma or (ileostoma) is a surgically created opening in the abdominal wall through which a small piece of the small intestine (ileum) or ureter is guided outwards onto the skin surface.

The stool or urine is excreted from the body through this artificially created opening instead of through the anus or ureter. There are several types of stoma, the most frequent type is the Colostoma

(stoma of the large intestine). There are two other types of stoma: the ileostoma (small intestine stoma) and the urostoma (stoma for urinary diversion). Other names for stoma are: "Artificial exit", "lateral exit", or "anus praeter."

The stoma itself is similar in appearance to the oral mucosa. It has a round or oval shape and can vary in size. Since the mucous membrane of the stoma has no nerve endings, touching the stoma is also not painful. It bleeds slightly when touched, which is completely harmless.

"How would my person describe the typical position of an ileostoma?"

The skin around the stoma must be protected from direct contact with the ileostoma excreta. The excrements are rich in digestive enzymes and therefore very aggressive. They can therefore be very irritating to the skin. In the optimal case, the ileostoma therefore stands about 1.5-3 cm away from the abdominal wall. A well-functioning stoma system prevents the stool from being pressed under the base plate, e.g. the adhesive surface of the stoma supply. These aggressive excrements of the ileostoma can flow into the bag.

"Should one be asking oneself whether the frequency of the excretions can be controlled?", my own person must answer this question:

In an ileostoma, the frequency of excretions can hardly be controlled by diet. An ileostoma produces excreta at any time and very irregularly. It might be possible to influence the consistency of the excreta to some extent.

"How can you get a firmer stool?"

Well, by including stuffing foods in one's diet. For example, bananas or potatoes areregularly consumed. Please always remember that the more liquid the excreta is, the more frequently the bag of the stoma supply must be emptied afterwards. Continence is lost through an ostomy system.

"What is continence?"

Continence is the ability to control stool and urine, and to control yourself when you go to the toilet. Some special supply systems have been developed to compensate for these disadvantages. Components are: A skin protection and a pouch. Skin protection prevents the stoma from being attacked by stool or urine. This is achieved by collecting the odour-tight excreta in a bag. Until the contents of the bag are disposed of in a toilet.

"Who gets a stoma?"

They are often relatively young people who wear stoma. Patients with chronic inflammatory bowel disease (CED), ulcerative colitis and Crohn's disease are often affected.

In the case of the diseases I have mentioned, it may well be necessary to switch off an inflamed section of the intestine for some time. So that this intestinal section can recover from the inflammation.

Familial adenomatous polyposis (hereditary intestinal cancer) often leads to a terminal ileostoma. In order to avoid a malignant course, the colon is completely removed in quite young people. Further causes for a temporary or terminal ileost are: Accidents, colon cancer and congenital malformations.

"Why a stoma?"

A stoma represents an extreme break in the life of every affected person. The stoma changes one's own body image. One no longergoes to the toilet normally, and the control over one's own excrements is partly lost.

When a life-threatening situation makes it necessary, surgeons create a stoma. An example of this could be: The removal of a colon cancer tumour that is so unfavourable that the anus and sphincter muscle must also be removed.

The surgeon would immediately be forced to guide the intestine to another location. And he creates a terminal stoma.

"But what does terminal mean ?"

It means that the stoma remains and cannot be removed again. There are patients who have Crohn's disease or colitis, for example. ulcerosa. These diseases manifest themselves mainly in violent and bloody Diarrhea.

In a large proportion of patients, the symptoms ofthe disease cannot be treated with medication, or only inadequately.

The consequence of this is that they are very limited in their everyday life and in their profession.

Here a stoma can provide a great relief that not every thought revolves around where the next toilet is.

The quality of life is temporarily or permanently improved by a stoma. Experience shows that older people are less able to cope with the new situation than younger people. Changes bring a certain restlessness into the previous life.

Chapter 4.

The stoma care and the ileostma: The excretions from an ileostoma are thin to thinly pulpy. The excretion volume is approximately 1.5 litres per day. Unfortunately, no stoma bag can absorb this amount. The weight would also pull unpleasantly on the filled pouch and thus on the abdomen.

Therefore, the supply with a so-called "open bag" is often realized. This "open bag" is often also called a stripping bag, it has an opening at the end. Through this opening the liquid to mushy content of the bag is emptied in the toilet. Afterwards the outlet is sealed absolutely tightly by a clamp or a velcro fastener. The change of a stoma: After a stoma operation, each patient is trained by trained stoma therapists, nurses or nurses in the handling of stoma care and the change of care. In theory, it is best to change the stoma care while standing or sitting in front of the sink. In practice, a change of stoma care in bed has proven to be very advantageous.

For example, if you are physically weak or have lost too much weight through several operations, you should first try in bed. In bed a Malör can also happen, there are enough templates for this unfavourable case. The preparation for a change of supply is as follows: First of all, all necessary materials have to be prepared. This includes especially cloths and non-sterile compresses, for cleansing the skin.

 Disposal of used stoma supplies: A new base plate and a new stoma bag including closure clip. If necessary, cut out the hole in the skin protection plate to fit.

After the stoma plate has been glued, no skin should be exposed around the stoma. A standard nail scissor is used to cut out the plate. A small garbage bag to remove the used stoma supply. In our example, stripping bags are used; these should be emptied in the toilet before removal.

Then the skin protection plate is removed from the skin from top to bottom. It might be helpful to press lightly against the abdomen above the supply. So that the skin is not lifted too much. The used treatment is disposed of in the rubbish bag provided. The bin liner should then be closed with a knot. This immediately ensures that there is no unpleasant odour nuisance.

In addition one should worry about the cleaning of the skin.

Cleaning the skin: The skin should now be cleaned of stool residues and residues of the skin protection plate. For this purpose, non - sterile compresses and various cleaning agents are often recommended. Strictly speaking, a cleansing with water would be sufficient in most cases. It is also the most beautiful variant at the same time. For the removal of remainders of the skin protection plate which cannot be removed with water alone, the use of plaster removers is recommended.

Since not every health insurance company covers the recommended compresses, it is also possible to replace them with disposable washcloths, firm toilet paper or kitchen paper can be used.

Exclude the use of normal washcloths and sponges. This would cause germs to form and eventually lead to infections. A washing additive that is pH-neutral is recommended for cleaning. Oil-containing cleaning lotions should not be used as they have a greasing effect.

The durability of the skin protection plate would be strongly, impaired in such a case. After cleaning, the skin should be well dried again.

Showering, bathing and swimming: Contact with water is not a problem for stoma care.

The stoma bag and the base plate are designed in such a way that they adhere safely and even equipped with a so-called activated carbon filter. This filter should be masked before contact with water. Small stickers are supplied with the stoma bags. By masking, the filter cannot be soaked with water and become clogged.

After swimming or showering, the stickers can be removed afterwards again, the filters function reliably to the stomach even in chlorine and salt water. Many stoma bags are immediately as usual.

On the other hand, stoma bags covered with fleece absorb water like a full cloth. But if you have a two-part supply system, changing the wet stoma bag is no problem at the end.

Another possibility would be to dry the wet stoma bag carefully afterwards with a towel or a hair dryer. It is also possible to simply remove the wet fleece carefully from the bag. Swimming with stoma: Swimming is even recommended for stoma wearers.

The body is evenly loaded and trained during swimming. There is also no excessive strain on the abdomen.

With a slightly higher cut swimsuit (bathing shorts), men can make their stoma care virtually disappear. Women, on the other hand, can hide their stoma care behind a swimsuit.

Showering and bathing is basically possible without stoma care. However, one should also do without moisturizing, oily bath additives and shower creams. Unfortunately, these have the characteristic to impair the adhesion of the base plates powerfully.

Chapter 5.

Partnership, family and friends. When you are confronted with an ostomy for the first time, you often ask yourself the following question:

"How will the family, one's own children and next of kin react to the stoma?"

„Should I even tell my friends about the stoma?" "Or should I hide it?"

"Will my friends react positively to the stoma?", "or should I turn away?"

We humans are all very different and therefore different, but also the reactions when they react with a taboo subject (stoma) of our society.

Of course, it is not possible to give general tips on how to behave towards friends andacquaintants at this point. Just deal openly with your "problem stoma" Partnership: After a stoma operation, many people feel unattractive and perhaps even a little disfigured by the many scars and the bag on their stomach. Even if the stoma was the life-saving way out, or at least the end of a long path of suffering.

„Can it be difficult at first to accept the change of one's own body?"

The faster one accepts the stoma, the easier it is to open oneself up to one's partner and then to deal with the new situation without any compulsion. A strengthened relationship nothing knocks over so fast, not even an ostomy. A partner will certainly worry more about you, the stoma only plays a minor role at first. It is important to talk openly with your partner about your own fears. Many relationships become stronger through the joint processing of such exceptional situations as illness and stoma surgery.

Children: Children deal with the subject of stoma very impartially and without prejudice. Children are very curious and often want to know what kind of bag is on their stomach and what it is good for. Children chat to third parties immediately, but they also like what comes to their mind. Children also want to know why dad or mum go to the hospital now. You should only tell the children so much about how you think you are right.

In doing so, also address their questions. You can talk openly about stoma surgery with somewhat older children. Just like their own partner, they are naturally worried and want to be informed about what will happen to them.

Friends and acquaintances: In most cases, friends and acquaintances are the first to know about a hospital stay. But what you tell them about a stoma is left to you. You should tell your next of kin if you consider the stoma to be part of your own privacy. Want to keep control over who you tell about your surgery and who you don't.

Many patients go through a positive experience, the positive reaction of friends and relatives, after they learned about the stoma. There is often astonishment that one does not even look at the disability. That someone but who turns away from a stoma is rather the absolute exception.

Sexual life with a stoma: From a medical point of view, a stoma is no reason for renouncing a fulfilled sexual life. For the special moments, the stoma can be discreetly supplied with opaque mini bags or stoma caps. In addition, bag covers made of fabric are offered, which make the contact of the bags with the skin pleasant. Emptying the bag before sexual activity should be a matter of course. There are some stoma wearers who have designed lingerie and underwear that make the stoma bag disappear in intimate moments, almost invisibly. These are available through Internet shops that have been set up specifically for this purpose.

Women as well as men may reject sexual activity after stoma surgery. The people affected fall victim to often difficult to accept her altered physical situation. They no longer feel attractive enough and dirty. A sensitive life partner who shows that you are still lovable and attractive even after the operation often works wonders in this difficult situation for the patient with a little patience.

You should not be afraid to seek medical or psychological help for this problem. Nutrition: The most discussed topic among stoma carriers is probably nutrition. People are often asked about special diets or some valuable tips.

But one thing anticipates my humble self, there is no special diet for stoma carriers. Basically, there are no dietary restrictions after the creation of a stoma. What was tolerated before the operation is also tolerated afterwards. Exceptions are special

Diets that have to be followed due to illnesses such as diabetes or after the removal of large parts of the small intestine.

Restrictions in diet due to constrictions and adhesions. If, however, there are basically no restrictions in the diet after a stoma!

"But why do so many sufferers report the intolerance of certain foods?"

After eating individual foods, complaints suchas stomach pain, cramps, lack of defecation or even vomiting are often reported.

Causes for these complaints are often so-called constrictions (stenoses) at the passage of the stoma on the stomach, or adhesions, clamps or adhesions. A constriction could occur directly at the stoma due to scarring. Adhesions are also consequences of the

Abdominal surgery. In most cases, complaints caused by adhesions occur in patients with an ileostoma.

In the case of a colostoma, they lead to complaints less frequently. This tendency to adhesions varies from patient to patient.

Many patients do not notice their slight adhesions and have no restrictions in their diet.

Other patients, on the other hand, suffer so much from the adhesions that they are severely restricted in their diet. Hardly digestible foods can stick to existing adhesions, or stenoses at the narrow places of the intestine, and cause colic-like complaints, up to the intestinal obstruction. In case of severe pain with vomiting, a doctor should be consulted.

"But how do you determine what you cannot tolerate?"

Particularly in the first weeks after an operation, individual intolerances become noticeable. It can be helpful to keep a nutrition diary. In this diary you record what you have eaten and when you have eaten something, as well as the symptoms that occur.

This makes it easy to identify any incompatibilities and how to design the diet afterwards. At this point it should be mentioned that very few foods are permanently intolerable.

"How do you eat correctly?"

A very important point is one's own eating habits. Less what, but how. Decisive for it is, how many different food one tolerates. Tips on eating behaviour: Eat slowly and chew. Chewing and chewing again, the better the food is crushed around, so easier the passage through the intestine falls.

Those affected should therefore take their time while eating, enjoy the food and chew well for a long time. Drink enough to eat, a large glass of water, preferably without carbonic acid. Avoid long-fibre, hard-shelled vegetables and fruits.

Small regular meals, five smaller meals a day. Sufficient exercise, depending on physical condition, half an hour walk. Experiences with Stomatsträger show, by a consistent conversion of the eating habits, existingcomplaints strongly to go back, and in addition still nearly all food are tolerated.

Flatulence: Each concerning with an artificial intestinal outlet (large or small intestine) experienced it already. At an unfavourable moment, all those present can clearly hear air coming out of the stoma.

"How should an affected person deal with it now? and how can such a situation be avoided?"

This is a completely natural process when gases form during digestion. These cannot be suppressed. It can become embarrassing when the air, in a meeting with work colleagues, birthday coffee, or in the cinema, looks for the way outside.

The formation of gases can be influenced by a conscious diet. Excessive consumption of fibre-rich foods promotes the formation of flatulence. My recommendation: herbal teas with anise, ginger, fennel, caraway and mint, against flatulence. Avoid all legumes completely or at least reduce them considerably. For carbonated drinks, the same applies as for legumes, since the carbon dioxide contained in the drink is responsible for the subsequent flatulence.

Bottom Line

If you are now one of those people who have been diagnosed with Crohn's disease, you should never give up. And yes, this diagnosis is a shock.

I also know exactly how you feel now, because I share the same fate with you. My person also knows that you are talking about a disease that cannot be cured. In spite of everything, one must try to cope with this illness. You can also get very old with Crohn's disease if you follow certain rules.

One of those people who have decided not to give up should fight now. It will be an eternal fight and the end is still completely open. Of course there will be beautiful and less beautiful days, progress and setbacks.

Learn from others and accept any help you can get. Alone you will most likely fail.

My person has been fighting for more than 17 years and has had a lot of help. Ours also experienced a lot of ups and downs. The knowledge from it:

The Crohn is asleep, but he can become active again (awake) at any time. After a hard time there is always a good time.

Life could be much easier, but unfortunately it is not.

Deal openly with the illness, don't pretend and don't hide here. This stress would save my own person from the beginning. Please think about it, the better your body is, the better it will be for yourselves. Therefore paybetter attention on you and on your bodies.

Giving up was for me personally, never a real

option! And exactly the same wishes for you, my person. Not to give up and to resign immediately at the first resistance, to despair or even to resign. Please don't do that!

At this point our (my) little story ends.

The End.

Acknowledgement

Although writing a book is often a lonely undertaking, no author can do without help. Every time one of my books appears, I stand in the foreground as an author. This is not particularly fair, because it always requires many people who make such a publication possible in the first place. That was of course also the case with me.

And all the dear people who have been a help to me during the writing, shall now find a special mention here. First of all I would like to thank my publisher BoD (Books on Demand). That anyone at all was willing to publish that was created by me, the motivating words when I was sitting in front of a blank page again and didn't know what to do. Thank you for the effort and patience, my much appreciated publisher (BoD).

And of course my thanks also go to my family, my parents, my brother and my three sisters. They have always given me the strength and time to devote to my book project. Without you I would never have been able to do that.

Wolfgang(S), Marzena(W) and Brigitte from Hamburg also have no small part in the completion.

Whenever I was about to throw everything in, you rebuilt me and encouraged me to continue.

Many thanks also to my readers and the future readers, you are one of the reasons why I write. Many Thanks to all also to those who were not mentioned by name. I appreciate that very much. Thank you.

Bibliography

Own history

Internet

Imprint (German)

J.R Lucas Wolf

luquetejero@hotmail.com

Print and Publishing: BoD - Books on Demand,
Norderstedt

Paperback ISBN: 978-3-7494-6779-2

Printed: In Germany

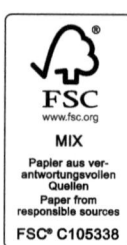